Vitamin Water Recipes: Quick & Easy Homemade Vitamin Drinks Made From Fruits & Vegetables

Ginger Langley

Copyright Information

Vitamin Water Recipes: Quick & Easy Homemade Vitamin Drinks Made from Fruits & Vegetables

Copyright © 2014 by Ginger Langley.

Skagit Books
http://skagitbooks.com

Photo Credit:
All interior photos copyright © 2014 Candace Sinclair
http://candacesinclairphotography.com

Accuracy Department—To my friends and business partners, I welcome any comments about errors or misprints you find in my book. Just email me at: gingerlangley1@gmail.com. Your assistance in helping me excel is highly valued.

Printed in the United States of America

Healthy Lifestyle Series, Book 1
First Edition: January 2014
Second Edition: November 2014

ISBN-13: 978-1496146151
ISBN-10: 1496146158

Contents

Disclaimer

The recipes and information provided in this book are not intended to replace the advice and recommendations from a medical professional or nutritionist regarding your health, diet, and eating habits.

If you try any of the recipes contained in this book, or act on the information provided, just know that you do so at your own risk. This author has taken every positive step and precaution to provide you with the most accurate information from her own recipe files.

Introduction

The idea for *Vitamin Water Recipes* was created out of my search for ways to consume more water during the day, so I could adequately maintain my health and hydrate my body.

Although I learned through reading various government publications that after drinking any beverage, it is necessary to follow up with an equal-sized quantity of water, it became a constant struggle for me when trying to drink eight glasses of water a day.

Doctors say that the amount of water in ounces that anyone should consume in one day should equal half of your body weight. For example, if you weigh 150 pounds, then your water intake for one day should be between 75-90 ounces. Wow! That's a lot of water, considering that a gallon of water accounts for 64 ounces.

To make this task more pleasurable, and since I was cutting back on tea and coffee beverages due to them taxing the acidity levels in my body, one morning, I boiled a mug of water and added a sprig of fresh mint, muddled to extract the mint flavor. My homemade beverage was quickly consumed.

Later in the day, I decided to add one-half of a sliced lemon, a slice of fresh ginger, and another sprig of mint to a heated cup of water. Yum! That's when I knew I'd better keep track of all this.

That same evening, I retrieved quart-sized canning jars from the top shelf of my pantry, determined to create four quarts of fruit and vegetable-infused water for consumption the next day. I muddled the ingredients to extract the most flavor, and then I added a handful of ice cubes on top of the ingredients and finally topped off each jar with filtered drinking water. I made sure to allow a half-inch clearance before sealing the jar with a lid and placing the jar in the refrigerator.

The next day, I easily drank four quarts of the vitamin water I had prepared the previous evening. With notepad in hand, I researched the vitamin and health benefits of each fruit and vegetable that I had combined to create a quart of vitamin water. I was pleasantly shocked at the nutritional and healing properties contained in each ingredient.

After you make up a batch or two of vitamin water and store it in your refrigerator for the next day, you'll quickly learn which flavors are your favorites. Also, you might not have all the ingredients on hand when you initially prepare your vitamin waters, and that's okay. Just combine the types of fruits, vegetables, and herbs that you like the best. If, for example, you don't have (or like) fresh mint or dill, you can omit the herb, and you'll still be able to enjoy a tasty and healthy vitamin water drink.

How long can I keep vitamin water in my refrigerator?

Vitamin water can remain in your refrigerator for approximately two days. I would not recommend storing it for a third day, since most of the ingredients would begin to turn bad, and therefore would become ineffective for maintaining your healthy lifestyle.

Which ingredients require muddling?

To derive the best vitamin value, I recommend muddling all herbs and all berries. For example, mint is most effective after it's muddled. Blueberries, cranberries, and raspberries are best when they're muddled.

After you've sampled and tasted various vitamin water recipes, you will begin to develop your own personal preferences for the ingredients you choose to include in your mixtures. For example, if you don't like the strong taste of muddled mint, then maybe reduce the amount of mint leaves you use, or else, don't muddle all the mint and then you'll still get all the vitamin benefits but will taste only a slight amount of mint flavor.

How long must the vitamin water be refrigerated before I can drink it?

You can drink your vitamin water after it's been refrigerated for a minimum of three hours. I recommend 12 hours or overnight to get the most benefit from the fruits, vegetables and herbs.

In the next section, I'll give you a list of utensils that you might find helpful if you decide to make your own vitamin water on a daily basis. Remember, it takes only a minute or two to make a quart of vitamin water, and it's much more cost effective and healthy than buying pre-made beverages. Plus, you get to regulate the quantity and taste of each beverage you prepare.

What should I do with the ingredients in the jar after drinking all the vitamin water?

You can dispose of the ingredients you placed in your one-quart jar, or you can use one or more of the ingredients in a smoothie, sorbet, or juice. Remember, these are still fresh ingredients, and as long as you keep them chilled or add them to a beverage in your high-speed blender, you'll be getting double the value for the price you paid for these healthy ingredients. It's your choice if you want to toss the ingredients or repurpose them into a healthy beverage, sauce, or snack.

WARNING: If you know you are allergic to a specific ingredient listed in a vitamin water recipe, then either omit the ingredient or else don't make the vitamin water. When in doubt, please check with a medical professional or a nutritionist who is familiar with your dietary restrictions.

NOTE: Some vitamin water recipes may contain additional ingredients that are not listed in the title of the vitamin water.

Optional Utensils

The utensils mentioned below are not a requirement for making homemade vitamin water, but these little gadgets are quite helpful.

Muddler. This is a type of stick that you use to tamp down the herbs, fruits, and vegetables when they're placed inside the jar to extract more of their oils, vitamins, and flavor. You can also use a wooden spoon.

> **Types of muddlers to buy.** You'll find wooden muddlers and stainless steel muddlers for sale at local stores or online. Either type of muddler will work perfectly as long as the end of the muddler is rounded and not rough; otherwise, it will shred your herbs or fruits, which isn't desirable.

Handheld sieve strainer. This is a little gadget that you might already have in your kitchen. You'll definitely want to strain the vitamin water before pouring it into your glass or mug.

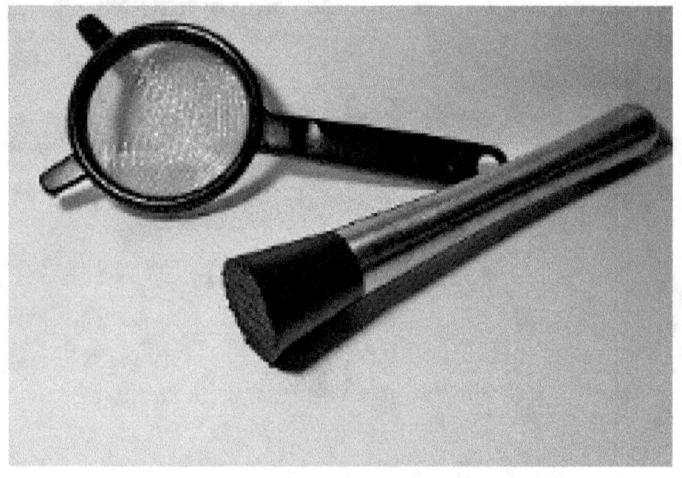

Handheld strainer (top) and muddler (bottom)

Plastic funnel. I use this inexpensive plastic funnel to help when I'm pouring my vitamin water into a drinking glass. The little strainer fits easily onto the top of the funnel, which makes it easy to get the water in the glass while the strainer traps the fruits, vegetables, or herbs from dropping into the water. Below are two views of the funnel.

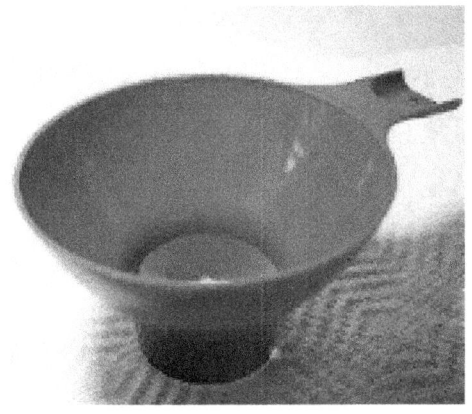

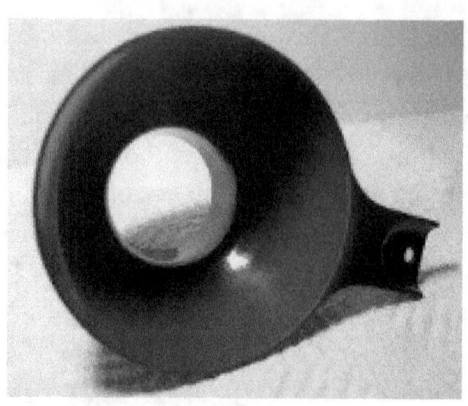

Funnels easily fit over a drinking glass and can
accommodate a small
handheld strainer on top.

Wide-mouth strainer. This type of strainer sells for
about $5 on Amazon, and it fits securely over a wide-
mouth canning jar, which makes it truly easy for not
getting seeds, bits of stalks, veggies, or herbs in your
vitamin water.

Wide-mouth 32-oz. or 16-oz. glass jars with lids. You
can purchase glass jars from almost any grocery store or
hardware store that's local to you. You can also save
money by ordering several cases of jars in quantity
through many online vendors.

If you are a thrift store shopper or you like to see what's available at garage sales, you can usually find canning jars for sale at reasonable prices. Then, all you would have to do is buy a package of lids and seals.

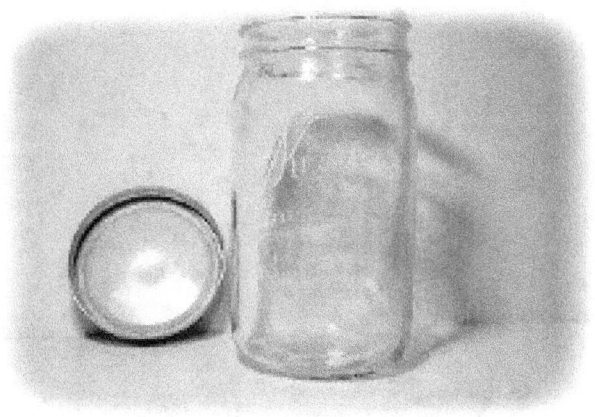

One-quart glass canning jar with lid

Ice cube trays (optional). If you have an icemaker that does a good job of making ice quickly, you probably won't need additional ice cube trays. But for me, personally, if I'm making four quart jars of vitamin water at one time and have to fill up every jar with ice cubes, I quickly use up most of the ice in my freezer compartment. That's why I have extra ice cube trays to keep up with the demand for ice cubes when making my vitamin water. Plastic ice cube trays are also available from grocery stores, and they are inexpensive.

VITAMIN WATER RECIPES

I've listed all the vitamin water recipes in alphabetical order, so it's easier for you to find the recipes that become your favorites.

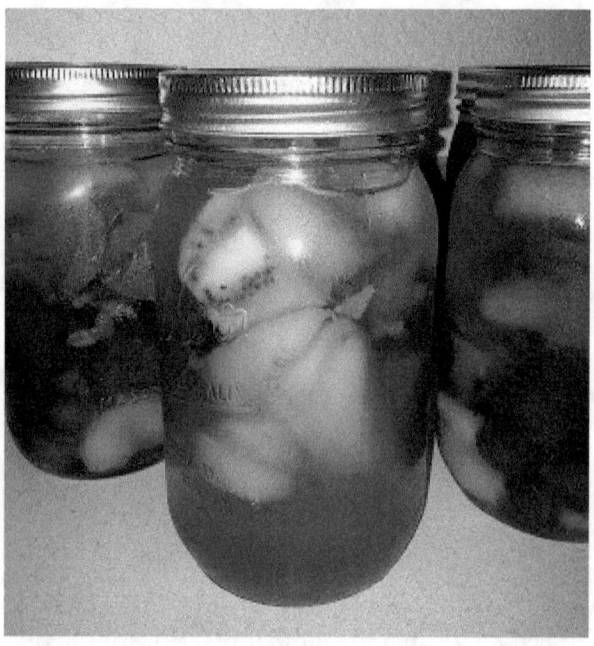

Three one-quart jars filled with vitamin water
ingredients ready to go into the refrigerator.

Apple and Cinnamon Vitamin Water

Although this vitamin water has only two ingredients in addition to the water and ice cubes, it's an easy-to-drink beverage that also tastes good as a hot beverage.

Ingredients

1 red apple, peeled and cut into chunks

1 cinnamon stick, whole (not powdered cinnamon, since it won't dissolve properly)

Filtered water

Ice cubes

Directions

Place the apple chunks and the cinnamon stick into the jar. Add a handful of ice cubes, and then fill the remainder of the jar with filtered water. Allow about one-half inch of space in the jar before sealing it.

Refrigerate your vitamin water overnight so the flavors have time to infuse the water and then served chilled.

If you're in a hurry to drink a glass of your vitamin water, allow at least three hours for it to chill in the refrigerator.

If you're dieting, this vitamin water can help to replace
nutrients and vitamins in your diet or replace one
calorie-laden snack.

Health Benefits

Apples have so many claims to health fame that people
seeking good health probably ignore what they were told
growing up. I know that the health and nutrition
properties in apples are a *vital* part of my daily diet,
and here's why. Apples help you avoid getting
Alzheimer's disease, and they protect you from
Parkinson's disease. They reduce tooth decay and
bacteria in your mouth.

Apples reduce the risk of getting pancreatic cancer by up
to 23 percent. They reduce your chances of getting
diabetes, they reduce your bad cholesterol levels, and
they make you have a healthier heart. They prevent the
formation of gallstones. They help you not get
constipated, but they also help if you get diarrhea.
(That's a miracle. because it works in both
directions…kind of like a Thermos bottle.)

Apples neutralize your system if you have irritable
bowel syndrome, and they ward off hemorrhoids.
Apples help to control your weight, they boost your
immune system, help prevent cataracts, and they
detoxify your liver.

Cinnamon is like one of those unbelievable spices that not only tastes good sprinkled on fruit, in smoothies, in coffee, and infused in hot water for a tasty beverage on a cold winter night, but cinnamon has so many healing and health benefits that it might make you want to sit up and pay attention when you learn more about it (which is why I put it in this vitamin water recipe).

Cinnamon lowers cholesterol, regulates your blood sugar, prevents cancer, stops yeast infections that even medicine can't help with, brings arthritis relief, is anti-bacterial, improves your brain functions, and makes blood anti-clotting, fights E. coli bacteria, and is high in nutrients.

Apple, Blueberry, Lemon, and Mint Vitamin Water

It doesn't matter what season it is, I always have these four ingredients in my kitchen. The antioxidant levels found in these fruits and the mint are helpful for maintaining a strong immune system.

I've tried substituting granny smith apples, but my preference is for any type of red apple.

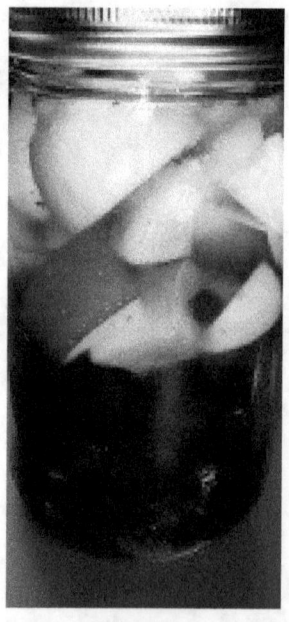

Apples, Blueberries, and Lemon Vitamin Water in a one-quart glass jar.

Ingredients

1 red apple, peeled and cut into chunks

1/2 cup blueberries (rinsed), fresh or thawed from frozen

1/2 lemon, cut in half, not peeled

5 mint leaves (just the leaves, not the stems)

Ice cubes

Filtered water

Directions

If you don't like the taste of mint, then omit the mint leaves.

In the bottom of a 1-quart glass jar, add the blueberries and mint leaves. Muddle them to extract the flavors and slightly bruise the blueberries.

Squeeze the pieces of lemon, and then add to the jar.

Add the apple chunks.

Add a handful of ice cubes and then fill the jar with water, but allow about one-half inch of space before sealing the jar and putting it in the refrigerator.

These vitamin water recipes are best when made the night before you intend to drink the water. However, the water will be infused with the healthy properties of the fruits, vegetables, and herbs after approximately three hours.

Health Benefits

Apples have so many claims to health fame that people seeking good health probably ignore what they were told growing up. I know that the health and nutrition properties in apples are a *vital* part of my daily diet, and here's why. Apples help you avoid getting Alzheimer's disease, and they protect you from Parkinson's disease. They reduce tooth decay and bacteria in your mouth. They reduce the risk of getting pancreatic cancer by up to 23%. They reduce your chances of getting diabetes, they reduce your bad cholesterol levels, and they make you have a healthier heart. They prevent the formation of gallstones. They help you not get constipated, but they also help if you get diarrhea. (That's a miracle. because it works in both directions…kind of like a Thermos bottle.)

Apples neutralize your system if you have irritable bowel syndrome, and they ward off hemorrhoids. Apples help to control your weight, they boost your immune system, help prevent cataracts, and they detoxify your liver.

Blueberries provide vitamin C and antioxidants. Also known to improve memory, they have a favorable impact on blood sugar regulation in persons already diagnosed with type 2 diabetes. In addition, blueberries contain vitamin K, manganese, fiber, and copper.

Lemons provide antibacterial, antiviral, and immune-boosting vitamins; they help with digestion, and they're a great liver cleanser. In addition, lemons also contain citric acid, pectin, bioflavonoids, vitamin C, magnesium, and limonene that help fight infection.

Mint leaves are known to reduce pain, to help with digestion of fats, and to soothe and calm the stomach. In addition, besides providing fantastic antioxidant qualities, mint contains menthol, which provides your body with a natural decongestant, breaking up mucus and phlegm. Mint is also known to help when you suffer from allergies during spring and fall. Recent health studies have indicated that mint is an effective treatment for anyone who has irritable bowel syndrome (IBS).

Apple, Cucumber, Basil, and Cinnamon Vitamin Water

This is my most prized vitamin water recipe that I drink every day to help me stay healthy. You might look at this list of ingredients and wonder what it would taste like. So, if you're skeptical, just make a one-quart jar of it. I happen to really like it.

My only warning with this vitamin water is that it's really only good for two days in your refrigerator, because the apple starts turning brown on the third day. But when you look at the health benefits, you might understand why I have incorporated this vitamin water into my daily favorites. That's why I have to make at least two jars every day just to keep the supply current.

Ingredients

1 cinnamon stick, whole (not powdered cinnamon, since it won't dissolve properly)

1 red apple, peeled and sliced thick

6 fresh basil leaves, muddled

1/2 cup cucumber, peeled and cubed

Filtered water

Ice cubes

Directions

Put the basil leaves into a one-quart glass jar and use a wooden spoon or a muddler to scrunch the leaves and get the vitamins and flavors working. Then add the cucumber, apple, and cinnamon stick.

Contrary to every other recipe in this book (except for the fennel-infused recipe), I like to add one-half cup warm-to-semi-hot water to this blend, and let it rest for about five minutes. Then fill the jar with ice cubes, and fill the remainder of the jar with room temperature water.

By adding the warm-to-hot water first and letting the mixture rest for a bit, it allows the cinnamon stick, the apple, and the basil to accelerate their flavor-producing qualities.

Store the jar in the refrigerator overnight, and taste your creation in the morning.

Health Benefits

Cinnamon is like one of those unbelievable spices that not only tastes good sprinkled on fruit, in smoothies, in coffee, and infused in hot water for a delish beverage on a cold winter night, but cinnamon has so many healing and health benefits that it might make you want to sit up and pay attention when you learn more about it (which is why I put it in this vitamin water recipe).

Cinnamon lowers cholesterol, regulates your blood sugar, prevents cancer, stops yeast infections that even medicine can't help with, brings arthritis relief, is anti-bacterial, improves your brain functions, and makes blood anti-clotting, fights E. coli bacteria, and is high in nutrients. Seriously, this vitamin drink is right up there with the best health benefits ever.

Basil is another sleeper herb, because it is so effective with improving your health, but unfortunately, some people just think it's used only for making Caprese (sliced tomatoes, sliced fresh mozzarella cheese, and basil doused with Balsamic vinegar and extra virgin olive oil) and nothing more. Basil is rich in beta-carotene that converts into Vitamin A and is a very powerful antioxidant. It improves your heart's health, prevents cancer, works as a moisturizer for skin and hair, treats acne and psoriasis, and is an anti-inflammatory food that heals and provides relief for anyone who has rheumatoid arthritis.

Basil keeps your digestive tract clean and healthy, keeps your bones and connective tissues strong, and it's classified as an anti-bacterial food. It improves your immune system and helps fight off those nasty viral infections like colds, herpes, and the flu. So, have you tried adding basil to your vitamin water lately?

Apples have so many claims to health fame that people seeking good health probably ignore what they were told growing up. I know that the health and nutrition properties in apples are a *vital* part of my daily diet, and here's why. Apples help you avoid getting Alzheimer's disease, and they protect you from Parkinson's disease. They reduce tooth decay and bacteria in your mouth. They reduce the risk of getting pancreatic cancer by up to 23%. They reduce your chances of getting diabetes, they reduce your bad cholesterol levels, and they make you have a healthier heart. They prevent the formation of gallstones. They help you not get constipated, but they also help if you get diarrhea.

Apples neutralize your system if you have irritable bowel syndrome, and they ward off hemorrhoids. Apples help to control your weight, they boost your immune system, help prevent cataracts, and they detoxify your liver.

Cucumbers are excellent for assisting with hydration, fighting cancer, skin care, blood pressure, teeth and gums, strong nails and hair, relieves arthritis pain, known to cure bad breath, good for those with diabetes, acts as a diuretic, helpful for weight loss, and for promoting hair growth.

Blueberries and Coconut Water

This handy two-ingredient recipe contains items that you can safely store in your freezer and pantry all year long. Blueberries can be purchased in bulk and frozen, and coconut water can be purchased fresh, kept in your refrigerator, or you can buy it in cans and containers and store it in your pantry.

With so many local stores selling coconut water and blueberries these days, it is easy to create a healthy vitamin water drink with these ingredients.

Ingredients

1/2 cup fresh or frozen blueberries

8-10 ounces coconut water

Ice cubes

Directions

Place 1/2 cup blueberries into a 1-quart glass jar, and muddle the blueberries to extract their healthy juices.

Add a handful of ice cubes.

Fill the glass jar with coconut water. The quantity of coconut water you'll need will depend upon how much room the blueberries use in the jar.

Seal the jar and place it in the refrigerator from three hours to overnight. Strain the fruit when you're ready to drink the vitamin water.

Health Benefits

Blueberries provide vitamin C and antioxidants. Also known to improve memory, and they have a favorable impact on blood sugar regulation in persons already diagnosed with type 2 diabetes. In addition, blueberries contain vitamin K, manganese, fiber, and copper.

Coconut water is not only a thirst quencher, but it helps in your efforts to lose weight. It also improves your hair, skin, and nails. It is good for settling your stomach and replacing electrolytes during those times when you're experiencing frequent urination and vomiting. Coconut water is known to increase the hydration levels in your body, lower your blood pressure, and it's rich in nutrients.

Blueberry, Cucumber, Lemon, and Mint Vitamin Water

Vitamin water is all the rage, but buying it in stores or online can be very expensive. If you're on a budget, you won't want to be paying those prices. This recipe is quick and easy, and you can save a lot of money by simply making your own vitamin water at home.

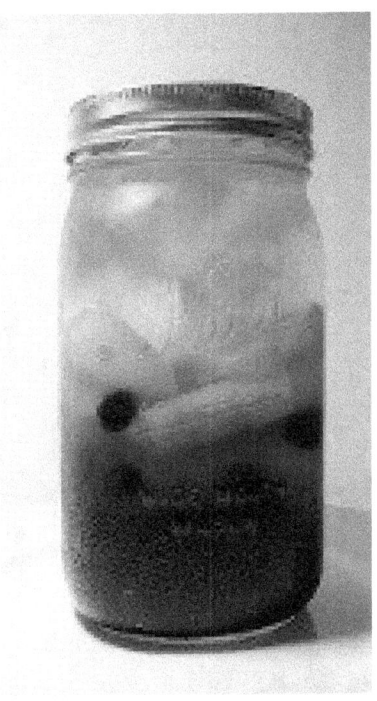

Blueberry, Cucumber, and Lemon Vitamin Water

Ingredients

1 cup slightly bruised (muddled) blueberries

6-8 thin slices of cucumber with peel left on

1 thinly sliced small lemon with peel left on

6 mint sprigs (to taste) slightly muddled

Filtered water

Ice cubes

Directions

Place slightly muddled blueberries into a one-quart glass jar. Now place the thinly sliced cucumber slices into the jar. Add in the thinly sliced lemon and the 6 mint sprigs, slightly bruised.

Pour the filtered water over the fruit, add a handful of ice cubes, and seal the glass jar with a lid. Make sure to allow about one-half inch of space between the ingredients and the lid.

Refrigerate your vitamin water overnight so the flavors have time to infuse the water and then served chilled. If you're in a hurry to pour a glass of your vitamin water, allow at least three hours for it to chill in the refrigerator.

If you're dieting, this vitamin water can help to replace nutrients and vitamins in your diet or replace one calorie-laden snack. Enjoy it as a refreshing beverage whenever you are thirsty or need to rehydrate.

Health Benefits

Blueberries provide vitamin C and antioxidants.

Cucumbers are excellent for assisting with hydration, fighting cancer, enhancing skin care, improving your blood pressure, teeth and gums, and they give you strong nails and hair, relieve arthritis pain, cure bad breath, and are good for anyone who has diabetes. Cucumbers act as a diuretic, are helpful for weight loss, and they're supposed to promote hair growth.

Lemons provide antibacterial, antiviral, and immune-boosting vitamins; they help with digestion, and they're a great liver cleanser. In addition, lemons contain citric acid, pectin, bioflavonoids, vitamin C, magnesium, and limonene that helps fight infection.

Mint leaves are known to reduce pain, to help with digestion of fats, and to soothe and calm the stomach.

Blueberry, Strawberry, Apple and Mint Vitamin Water

Berries and apple and mint...oh yay! This delicious combination of blueberries, strawberries, apple and mint leaves creates vitamin water that is not only nutritious and tasty, but it has so many healing properties that you just might want to add this recipe to your list of favorites.

What I like about this recipe combination is that the blueberries, strawberries, apples, and mint are available all year long. Apples and mint are always stocked in the fresh produce section of your grocery store, and bags of frozen strawberries and blueberries are located in the freezer aisle just ready for you to buy.

Even without the mint leaves, this fruit combo is delicious tasting, but if you do like the taste and healing qualities of mint, then you'll enjoy the added sweetness.

Ingredients

6 strawberries, cut in half (fresh or thawed from frozen)

1/2 cup blueberries (rinsed), fresh or thawed from frozen

1 small red apple, peeled and quartered

6-10 mint leaves (for a more subtle mint flavor, reduce the quantity of mint leaves)

Filtered water

Ice cubes

Directions

Place blueberries and mint leaves into a one-quart glass jar and muddle the berries and mint to extract their juices. Now place the strawberry and apple slices into the jar.

Add a handful of ice cubes, pour filtered water over the mixture, and then seal the glass jar with a lid. Make sure to allow about one-half inch of space between the ingredients and the lid.

Store in the refrigerator for up to two days before serving. Make sure to strain the fruit and mint leaves before pouring the vitamin water into your favorite drinking glass.

Health Benefits

Blueberries provide vitamin C and antioxidants. Also known to improve memory, and they have a favorable impact on blood sugar regulation in persons already diagnosed with type 2 diabetes. In addition, blueberries contain vitamin K, manganese, fiber, and copper.

Strawberries, regardless if they are fresh or frozen, contain iodine and antioxidants, such as Vitamin C, that prevents wrinkles, helps people with thyroid problems, and regulates your digestive system. Strawberries are an anti-inflammatory, known to prevent cancer and restore eyes to a healthy state, they boost your immune system, assist with the prevention of cardiovascular conditions, and improve the health of your bones.

Apples have so many claims to health fame that people seeking good health probably ignore what they were told growing up. I know that the health and nutrition properties in apples are a *vital* part of my daily diet, and here's why. Apples help you avoid getting Alzheimer's disease, and they protect you from Parkinson's disease. They reduce tooth decay and bacteria in your mouth. They reduce the risk of getting pancreatic cancer by up to 23 percent. They reduce your chances of getting diabetes, they reduce your bad cholesterol levels, and they make you have a healthier heart. They prevent the formation of gallstones. They help you not get constipated, but they also help if you get diarrhea.

Apples neutralize your system if you have irritable bowel syndrome, and they ward off hemorrhoids.

Apples help to control your weight, they boost your immune system, help prevent cataracts, and they detoxify your liver.

Mint leaves (muddled) are known to reduce pain, they help with digestion of fats, and they soothe and calm the stomach.

Cucumber, Orange, and Lemon Vitamin Water

Vitamin water is an ideal way to get a refreshing drink and some extra vitamins and minerals into your diet. It's easy and convenient to make at home, and you won't need a lot of expensive ingredients. Ideal for dieters, this refreshing drink can replace a calorie-heavy snack any time during the day as well as hydrate and provide the dieter with a feeling of being full, which helps curb hunger.

Ingredients

1 small cucumber sliced thin (do not peel)

1 small lemon sliced thin (do not peel)

4 thin slices of a Naval orange (do not peel)

Fresh mint sprigs, to taste (optional)

Filtered water

Ice cubes

Directions

Place the cucumber and orange slices into a clean 1-quart glass jar. Then add the lemon and mint. Drop in a handful of ice cubes. Add filtered water and then seal the jar with the lid and place the jar into the refrigerator overnight to chill.

In the morning, you'll have a jar of chilled vitamin water, ready to be strained and poured into a glass with ice that you can serve immediately. This is perfect to quench your thirst and hydrate your body.

Health Benefits

Lemons provide antibacterial, antiviral, and immune-boosting vitamins; they help with digestion, and they're a great liver cleanser. In addition, lemons also contain citric acid, pectin, bioflavonoids, vitamin C, magnesium, and limonene that helps fight infection.

Oranges provide nutrients like Vitamin C, A, and B1, beta carotene, pectin, folic acid, calcium, iron, manganese, chlorine and zinc. The antioxidant qualities of this citrus fruit are instrumental in preventing some types of cancer, lowering cholesterol, and high blood pressure, strengthening your immune system, easing arthritis, helping regulate the heart, and can keep sperm healthy so it is less likely to cause birth defects in the unborn child. Oranges help to prevent kidney stones, helps with weight loss, prevents ulcers, keeps your teeth and bones strong, and helps to relieve infections and constipation.

Mint leaves are known to reduce pain, to help with digestion of fats and to soothe and calm the stomach.

Cucumbers are excellent for assisting with hydration, fighting cancer, skin care, blood pressure, teeth and gums, strong nails and hair, relieves arthritis pain, known to cure bad breath, good for those with diabetes, a diuretic, helpful for weight loss, and they're good for promoting hair growth.

Dill, Cucumbers, and Pineapple Vitamin Water

I created this recipe quite a while ago just out of curiosity and because these ingredients were available in my refrigerator. It tasted good, and I decided to add it to my list of favorite vitamin waters.

The only thing I would suggest is to have some type of a fine mesh strainer handy before you pour the juice into your glass. Otherwise, the tiny dill fronds will swirl around in your water. I didn't want them lodging between my teeth, so I strained the mixture before pouring it into my traveling water bottle. Then I headed out the door ready for my morning hike. Of course, the tiny fronds won't hurt you. But if you're serving this vitamin water to a friend or family member, you might see their noses wrinkle if you don't strain the vitamin water before serving it.

Ingredients

Cucumber, about four inches sliced, not peeled, but scrubbed good to remove any residue wax

1 sprig of dill, uncut

1/2 lemon, cut in slices, not peeled

1 cup fresh pineapple, cut in big chunks

Filtered water

Ice cubes

Directions

Combine all ingredients into a quart-sized glass jar, fill with ice cubes, and then top off with filtered water. Seal the jar and place in the refrigerator for three hours or overnight.

Health Benefits

Cucumbers are excellent for assisting with hydration, fighting cancer, skin care, blood pressure, teeth and gums, strong nails and hair, relieves arthritis pain, known to cure bad breath, good for those with diabetes, acts as a diuretic, helpful for weight loss and hair growth.

Dill is such a delicate looking herb, but it packs a huge health punch, especially when its vitamins are released in water. It's good for osteoporosis, fighting off infections, protecting against free radicals, improving your digestion, soothing an upset stomach, and preventing diarrhea. It's also good as an instant remedy if you have hiccups, making headaches go away, calming your nerves, and helping you to sleep.

Lemons provide antibacterial, antiviral, and immune-boosting vitamins; they help with digestion and they're a great liver cleanser. In addition, lemons also contain citric acid, pectin, bioflavonoids, vitamin C, magnesium, and limonene that helps fight infection.

Pineapple, as you probably already know, is an excellent enzyme nutrient that helps you breathe better, improves the health of your heart, gets your blood circulation flowing better, improves your respiratory system, especially if you are prone to allergies or asthma, and on top of all this, it's also an anti-inflammatory. If you have ever had surgery, pineapple is this sort-of miracle fruit that eases trauma from incisions and is a great choice when you want to ease your pain if you have arthritis.

Fresh Fennel and Citrus Vitamin Water

In order to prepare fresh fennel and citrus vitamin water, you will need a 1-quart glass jar, filtered water, dried and crushed fennel, lemon juice, an orange, a few mint leaves, and a handful of ice cubes.

This vitamin water is rich in vitamin C and will help you digest your food. You can drink it to replace store-bought juices or as a vitamin supplement.

Ingredients

1 small orange, peeled, divided into segments, and sliced thin

3/4 teaspoon dried and crushed fennel

Juice of 1 small lemon (reserve peel to add to the water)

12 mint leaves, chopped (or less, if you prefer a more citrus taste)

Filtered water

Ice cubes

Directions

Start by boiling half a cup of water. Infuse between 1/4 to 3/4 teaspoonful of dried and crushed fennel and wait for the mixture to cool down.

Fill your glass jar with some cool water and add the water in which you infused the fennel. Extract the juice from the lemon and add it to the mix. You can also slice the leftover lemon and add it to your vitamin water to give it a richer citrus flavor.

Slice the orange as thinly as you can. Use a small orange or do not add all the slices to the mixture if you're working with a large orange.

You should then add twelve chopped mint leaves. You can add more or less mint depending on how much mint flavor you want or like. Mint leaves are rich in vitamins A and C, so adding more to the recipe makes it even healthier.

Place the glass jar in the refrigerator overnight so the vitamin water can chill.

Health Benefits

Lemons provide antibacterial, antiviral, and immune-boosting vitamins; they help with digestion and they're a great liver cleanser. In addition, lemons also contain citric acid, pectin, bioflavonoids, vitamin C, magnesium, and limonene that helps fight infection.

Oranges provide nutrients like Vitamin C, A, and B1, beta carotene, pectin, folic acid, calcium, iron, manganese, chlorine and zinc. The antioxidant qualities of this citrus fruit are instrumental in preventing some types of cancer, lowering cholesterol and high blood pressure, strengthening your immune system, easing arthritis, helping regulate the heart, and keeps sperm healthy so it is less likely to cause birth defects in the unborn child. Oranges help to prevent kidney stones, helps with weight loss, prevents ulcers, keeps your teeth and bones strong, and helps to relieve infections and constipation.

Mint leaves are known to reduce pain, to help with digestion of fats, and to soothe and calm the stomach.

Fennel assists with constipation, diarrhea, respiratory problems, indigestion, anemia, flatulence, menstrual problems, and it also helps improve your eyesight.

Ginger, Orange, and Mint Vitamin Water

Ginger and orange infused vitamin water is an excellent choice if you need to add more vitamins to your diet. Making your own vitamin water at home is actually a much healthier alternative to taking multi-vitamin supplements or to purchasing juices enriched with vitamins.

Ingredients

5 slices of fresh ginger, peeled, and not grated

1 small orange, divided into segments

5 mint leaves, chopped

One and one-half cups of filtered water

Ice cubes

Directions

You can make ginger-orange-mint vitamin water by pouring cool filtered water into the 1-quart glass jar.

Add the pieces of ginger, the orange segments, the mint leaves, and a handful of ice cubes.

Seal the jar with a lid and store the jar in the refrigerator overnight. This will give the ginger plenty of time to release its vitamins into the water. Your homemade vitamin water should stay good for a couple of days if you keep it sealed in a glass jar in the refrigerator.

Health Benefits

Mint leaves are known to reduce pain, to help with digestion of fats, and to soothe and calm the stomach.

Oranges provide nutrients like Vitamin C, A, and B1, beta carotene, pectin, folic acid, calcium, iron, manganese, chlorine and zinc. The antioxidant qualities of this citrus fruit is instrumental in preventing some types of cancer, lowering cholesterol and high blood pressure, strengthening your immune system, easing arthritis, helping regulate the heart, and keeps sperm healthy so it is less likely to cause birth defects in the unborn child. Oranges help to prevent kidney stones, helps with weight loss, prevents ulcers, keeps your teeth and bones strong, and helps to relieve infections and constipation.

Ginger is known to help protect men and women from cancer due to its antioxidant and anti-inflammatory health properties. If you've ever had indigestion or suffered from motion sickness, ginger is the natural remedy to take.

Lemon, Cucumber, and Rosemary Vitamin Water

This vitamin water recipe has strong flavors due to the citrus taste of the lemon and the fragrant aroma of fresh rosemary. The cucumber somewhat neutralizes the two stronger components of this recipe, and when combined, these three ingredients deliver a healthy punch to your consumption of water.

If for any reason, you do not like the fresh rosemary taste, you can substitute another herb that suits your palette. However, once you discover all the benefits of drinking a glass of water that contains rosemary, you'll be amazed at how this powerful herb can have a positive influence on your health.

Ingredients

1/2 lemon, sliced, unpeeled

6 spears of cucumber, each about 4-6 inches long

1 sprig of rosemary leaves, no stems (muddled to release nutritional properties)

Filtered water

Ice cubes

Directions

Place the rosemary into a 1-quart jar and muddle the herb to bring out the healthy vitamins and release them into the water. Add the cucumber spears, and the lemon.

Toss in a handful of ice cubes, and then fill the remainder of the jar with filtered water. Allow about one-half inch of space in the jar before sealing it.

Refrigerate your vitamin water overnight so the flavors have time to infuse the water and then served chilled.

Health Benefits

Lemons provide antibacterial, antiviral, and immune-boosting vitamins; they help with digestion, and they're a great liver cleanser. In addition, lemons also contain citric acid, pectin, bioflavonoids, vitamin C, magnesium, and limonene that helps fight infection.

Cucumbers are excellent for assisting with hydration, fighting cancer, for skin care, lowering blood pressure, keeping teeth and gums healthy, and growing strong nails and hair. Cucumbers are known to relieve arthritis pain, cure bad breath, are good for those with diabetes, and it acts as a diuretic, and is helpful for weight loss.

Rosemary is said to be a cancer-preventative herb. It's oftentimes used as a diuretic and for helping calm an upset stomach. Besides being so aromatic, it is also used as a sedative, and it has antispasmodic and antiseptic properties. If you suffer from fatigue or neuralgia, rosemary should be your go-to herb. The benefits of rosemary also include its ability to treat dizziness from many types of inner ear ailments. It's helpful for relieving headaches, reducing pain, and even helping to get rid of bad breath.

Lime and Raspberry Vitamin Water

Although this vitamin water has only two ingredients in addition to the water and ice cubes, it makes a thirst-quenching beverage that is loaded with antioxidants.

Ingredients

1 lime, rinsed well and cut into quarters (do not peel)

1/2 cup fresh or frozen raspberries (thawed)

Filtered water

Ice cubes

Directions

Place the raspberries into a 1-quart jar and muddle the fruit to bring out the healthy antioxidants and to infuse the juice into the water. Add the lime and a handful of ice cubes, and then fill the remainder of the jar with filtered water. Allow about one-half inch of space in the jar before sealing it.

Refrigerate your vitamin water overnight so the flavors have time to infuse the water and then served chilled.

Health Benefits

Limes are great as a thirst-quencher, and they contain more vitamin C than a lemon. When you're starting to fall asleep during the day, lime juice can help you stay alert and awake. It gets rid of those tired and can't-do-anything-today feelings from exhaustion and burnout.

Doctors often prescribe lime juice to patients to help them lower their blood cholesterol, to maintain healthy teeth, gums, and bones, and the vitamin C in a lime is known to help resist disease. The rind contains an oil that improves digestion. The juice of a lime helps with constipation, cataracts, and relieves peptic ulcers. Finally, lime juice is known to protect people from bacterial poisoning. For one small, green fruit, this citrus fruit sure delivers a multitude of health benefits.

Raspberries are loaded with so many nutrients, they're amazing! They help control free radicals that damage DNA cells, and raspberries are responsible for healthy weight loss, managing the immune system, vision, anti-aging, cancer, macular degeneration, heart health, iron deficiency, inflammation of the joints, diabetes, reducing nausea, and reducing pain for mothers during childbirth, because raspberries prevent hemorrhaging.

Orange and Basil-Infused Vitamin Water

At any time of the year, I usually have oranges and basil in my kitchen, so making this simple, two-ingredient vitamin water doesn't require a separate shopping trip. Since both ingredients provide vitamins crucial to maintaining a healthy body, this is often one of my go-to recipes.

Ingredients

4 thin slices of a Naval orange (do not peel)

6 fresh basil leaves, muddled

Filtered water

Ice cubes

Directions

Place the basil leaves into a 1-quart glass jar and with a muddler or wooden spoon, muddle the leaves to extract the basil's oil. Then add the orange slices. Toss in a handful of ice cubes and fill the jar with filtered water or tap water to within one-half inch of the opening. Seal the jar with a lid and place the jar into the refrigerator overnight to chill.

In the morning, you'll have a jar filled with chilled, delicious vitamin water. To serve, strain the contents into a drinking glass and serve immediately. This is perfect to quench your thirst and hydrate your body.

Health Benefits

Oranges provide nutrients like Vitamin C, A, and B1, beta carotene, pectin, folic acid, calcium, iron, manganese, chlorine and zinc. The antioxidant qualities of this citrus fruit are instrumental in preventing some types of cancer, lowering cholesterol and high blood pressure, strengthening your immune system, easing arthritis, helping regulate the heart, and keeps sperm healthy so it is less likely to cause birth defects in the unborn child. Oranges help to prevent kidney stones, helps with weight loss, prevents ulcers, keeps your teeth and bones strong, and helps to relieve infections and constipation.

Basil is an herb which is so effective for improving your health. It's rich in beta-carotene that converts into Vitamin A, and it's a very powerful antioxidant. It improves your heart's health, prevents cancer, works as a moisturizer for skin and hair, treats acne and psoriasis, and is an anti-inflammatory food that heals and provides relief for anyone who has rheumatoid arthritis.

Basil keeps your digestive tract clean and healthy, keeps your bones and connective tissues strong, and it's classified as an anti-bacterial food. It improves your immune system and helps fight off those nasty viral infections like colds, herpes, and the flu.

Peaches and Cucumber Vitamin Water

Even when peaches are not in season, I can always rely on my local grocery store to carry bags of frozen organic peaches, already sliced and ready to use. Sometimes when peaches are in season, I end up eating them before I can slice some into a glass jar for vitamin water, and that's okay. Regardless, peaches are always good at providing nutritional value and health benefits, however they are consumed.

In this recipe, I've combined peaches with slices of peeled cucumber to create a quick, two-ingredient vitamin water that's truly a pleasant-tasting beverage.

Ingredients

1/2 cup sliced peaches

1/2 small cucumber, peeled, and sliced into long spears

Filtered water

Ice cubes

Directions

Add the sliced peaches and cucumbers into a 1-quart glass jar. Toss in a handful of ice cubes, fill the jar with water, and seal. Place the jar in the refrigerator and allow three to twelve hours for the ingredients to fuse with the water.

When ready, strain the mixture by holding a small sieve over a drinking glass, and pouring the contents inside. Enjoy!

Health Benefits

Cucumbers are excellent for assisting with hydration, fighting cancer, for skin care, lowering blood pressure, keeping teeth and gums healthy, and growing strong nails and hair. Cucumbers are known to relieve arthritis pain, cure bad breath, are good for those with diabetes, and it acts as a diuretic, and is helpful for weight loss.

Peaches, low in calories, do not contain any saturated fats. They're packed with vitamins A, B, and C, which provide antioxidant benefits to your body when consumed in a solid or liquid state. Mineral-rich peaches are noted for their valuable levels of potassium, iron, and fluoride, which are what we need for healthy bones, teeth, heart rate, and blood pressure. Peaches also are great for slowing down the aging process and the onslaught of various diseases.

Pear-Ginger Vitamin-Infused Water

The pear-ginger vitamin water imparts several health benefits when you drink several glasses of it during the day. The sweetness of the pear helps to offset the strong flavor of the ginger. Yet, when combined and allowed to mellow overnight in your refrigerator, the taste is quite flavorful.

I realize that some of you may not like the taste of ginger, but if you're concerned about jump-starting a new regime of health benefits without any medical risks, you might want to try this vitamin water at least once. For those of us who like the combination of these flavors infused into a nutritious water beverage, you'll be surprised at how these two ingredients can easily be added to your regular shopping list.

Ingredients

1/2 of a fresh pear cut into chunks (do not peel)

Fresh ginger – 2 peeled slices for non-ginger lovers, or a one-inch knob, peeled and sliced thin if you want the ultimate health benefits

Filtered water

Ice cubes

Directions

Place the chunks of pear and all the ginger slices into a 1-quart glass jar. Muddle both ingredients. Add a handful of ice cubes, and then fill the jar with water before sealing it with a lid.

Place the jar in the refrigerator overnight. Strain the pear and ginger before pouring the vitamin water into a glass or mug.

Health Benefits

Pears are known to fight free radicals, they have a high content of vitamins K and C, and they act as an antioxidant that protects your cells and your heart. Since pears contain essential dietary fiber, they help to lower your bad levels of cholesterol. Besides all these awesome nutrition benefits, they can help anyone who might be susceptible to strokes, and pears have been mentioned in the medical community as being capable of helping to prevent cancer.

If you have been told to limit various types of fruits and vegetables due to their allergic reaction in your body, you might be happy to learn that pears are considered hypoallergenic, and are often included as the first fruit to give to infants.

If you're worried about the sugar content in fruits, pears are known to contain nutrients responsible for controlling diabetes, since they have such a low glycemic index. According to online charts, one pear has approximately 26 grams of carbs, and in this vitamin water recipe, we're using only one-half of a pear or about 13 grams. This means that pears can prevent blood sugar spikes.

The best prices for pears usually occur when they appear in the market from August to October. Just remember that pears, unlike other fruits, ripen from the inside, so do remember to check the thinnest part of the fruit before bringing it home to make sure it's still firm.

The reason I've listed this ingredient with its skin on is because there are so many powerful nutrients in the skin that it would be a shame to lose any of the healthy benefits of this fruit by peeling it.

Ginger is known to help protect men and women from cancer due to its antioxidant and anti-inflammatory health properties. If you've ever had indigestion or suffered from motion sickness, ginger is the natural remedy to take.

Pineapple and Cucumber Vitamin Water

This fruit and vegetable-infused beverage provides a multitude of vitamins and antioxidants that your body will love for all the health benefits. Not everyone will have fresh or frozen pineapple on hand, but for those times when you'd like a profound energy boost, this is the vitamin water to make.

Ingredients

3 slices of fresh pineapple or 1 cup of pineapple chunks

4-6 inch spears of thick-sliced cucumber, peeled

Filtered water

Ice cubes

Directions

Place the pineapple and cucumber slices into a 1-quart jar, muddling both ingredients to extract the juices and infuse the liquid into the water.

Add a handful of ice cubes, and then fill the jar with water before sealing it with a lid. Place it in the refrigerator overnight. Strain the pineapple and cucumber before pouring the vitamin water into a drinking glass or mug.

Health Benefits

Pineapple, as you probably already know, is an excellent enzyme nutrient that helps you breathe better, improves the health of your heart, gets your blood circulation flowing better, improves your respiratory system, especially if you are prone to allergies or asthma, and on top of all this, it's also an anti-inflammatory. If you have ever had surgery, pineapple is this sort-of miracle fruit that eases trauma from incisions and is a great choice when you want to ease your pain if you have arthritis.

Cucumbers are excellent for assisting with hydration, fighting cancer, for skin care, lowering blood pressure, keeping teeth and gums healthy, helpful for weight loss, and growing strong nails and hair. Cucumbers are known to relieve arthritis pain, cure bad breath, and are helpful for persons who have diabetes. Cucumbers also act as a diuretic.

Pomegranate, Cucumber, and Ginger Vitamin Water

You don't have to spend a lot of money on healthy vitamin water from the store. In fact, you can make it in the comfort of your own home with a few simple ingredients. Dieters and non-dieters alike will love Pomegranate Vitamin Water.

Ingredients

1 fresh pomegranate, seeded (or one cup frozen organic pomegranate seeds)

1 cucumber thinly sliced with skin on

1 one-inch knob of fresh ginger root

Fresh mint or rosemary sprigs (add herbs to suit your taste)

Ice cubes

Filtered water

Directions

Open and seed your pomegranate. (An average size pomegranate contains about 600 seeds.) You should have about one cup or more of seeds depending upon the size of your pomegranate. Lightly bruise the seeds with the side of your knife, a small rolling pin, or a muddler.

Put the seeds (about one cup or more to taste) in the jar. Add in the thinly sliced cucumber and the herbs of your choice and quantity. Add in the one-inch piece of fresh ginger root. (Important: Don't use powdered ginger, because it won't dissolve properly.)

Now pour the filtered water over your fruit in the jar to within one inch of the top. If using the rosemary or mint, add a few sprigs on the top. Then add a handful of ice cubes.

Seal the jar, place it in the refrigerator overnight, and serve chilled in the morning. Delicious.

Health Benefits

Cucumbers are excellent for assisting with hydration, fighting cancer, skin care, blood pressure, teeth and gums, strong nails and hair, relieves arthritis pain, known to cure bad breath, good for those with diabetes, a diuretic, helpful for weight loss, and promoting hair growth.

Ginger is known to help protect men and women from cancer due to its antioxidant and anti-inflammatory health properties. If you've ever had indigestion or suffered from motion sickness, ginger is the natural remedy to take.

Mint leaves are known to reduce pain, to help with digestion of fats, and to soothe and calm the stomach.

Rosemary is said to be a cancer-preventative herb. It's oftentimes used as a diuretic and for helping calm an upset stomach. Besides being so aromatic, it is sometimes used as a sedative and it has antispasmodic and antiseptic properties. If you suffer from fatigue or neuralgia, rosemary should be your go-to herb. But the benefits of rosemary also include its ability to treat dizziness from many types of inner ear ailments. It's helpful for relieving headaches, reducing pain, and even helping to get rid of bad breath.

Pomegranates are high in fiber, low in calories, high in vitamins and phytochemicals, and all this keeps your heart healthy. Plus, this fruit is known to prevent cancer. If you want to lose weight, pomegranate seeds have only 83 calories in about three-quarters of a cup.

Raspberry, Cucumber, and Lime Vitamin Water

If you're trying to lose weight, and you'd like to enjoy a delicious drink, look no further. This vitamin water is a great source of vitamins and an excellent thirst quencher. Simply replace one high calorie snack with some of this healthy raspberry vitamin water and you're well on the road to a healthier you.

Ingredients

One thinly sliced lime (do not peel)

One small cucumber thinly sliced (about 6 to 8 inches in total); do not peel but wash well.

1 cup slightly bruised (muddled) raspberries

Filtered water

Ice cubes

Directions

Place the thinly sliced lime, thinly sliced cucumber and the cup of raspberries into a 1-quart glass jar with the filtered water. Add a handful of ice cubes. Seal the jar and place it in the refrigerator overnight to chill.

Drink this in place of one snack each day while on your weight-loss plan.

This vitamin water drink is also great for rehydrating your body after a workout or a walk. Drink this in place of plain water or calorie laden snacks to help curb the appetite while dieting.

Full of healthy vitamins and antioxidants, this water is an ideal source for anyone who is trying to live a healthier lifestyle and wants to lose weight.

Health Benefits

Limes are great as a thirst-quencher, and they contain more vitamin C than a lemon. When you're starting to fall asleep during the day, lime juice can help you stay alert and awake. It gets rid of those tired and can't-do-anything-today feelings from exhaustion and burnout.

Doctors often prescribe lime juice to patients to help them lower their blood cholesterol, to maintain healthy teeth, gums and bones, and vitamin C is known to help resist disease. The rind contains an oil that improves digestion. The juice of a lime helps with constipation, cataracts, and relieves peptic ulcers. Finally, lime juice is known to protect people from bacterial poisoning. For one small, green fruit, this citrus fruit sure delivers a multitude of health benefits.

Raspberries are loaded with so many nutrients, they're amazing! They help control free radicals that damage DNA cells, and raspberries are responsible for healthy weight loss, managing the immune system, vision, anti-aging, cancer, macular degeneration, heart health, iron deficiency, inflammation of the joints, diabetes, reducing nausea, and reducing pain for mothers during childbirth, because raspberries prevent hemorrhaging.

Cucumbers are excellent for assisting with hydration, fighting cancer, skin care, blood pressure, teeth and gums, strong nails and hair, relieves arthritis pain, known to cure bad breath, good for those with diabetes, acts as a diuretic, helpful for weight loss, and for promoting hair growth.

Raspberry and Orange Vitamin Water

If you're trying to lose weight, and you'd like to enjoy a delicious drink, look no further. This vitamin water is a great source of vitamins and an excellent thirst quencher. Drink this in place of one snack each day while on your weight-loss plan.

This vitamin water drink is also great for rehydrating your body after a workout or a walk. Drink this in place of plain water or calorie-laden snacks to help curb the appetite while dieting.

Full of healthy vitamins and antioxidants, this water is an ideal source for anyone who is trying to live a healthier lifestyle and wants to lose weight.

Ingredients

1 cup slightly bruised (muddled) raspberries

1/2 orange, segments, halved (no pith or peel)

Filtered water

Ice cubes

Directions

Place the raspberries into a 1-quart jar and muddle the fruit to bring out the healthy antioxidants and to infuse the juice into the water. Add the orange slices and a handful of ice cubes, and then fill the remainder of the jar with filtered water. Allow about one-half inch of space in the jar before sealing it.

Refrigerate your vitamin water overnight so the flavors have time to infuse the water and then served chilled after straining the fruit.

Health Benefits

Raspberries are loaded with so many nutrients, they're amazing! They help control free radicals that damage DNA cells, and raspberries are responsible for healthy weight loss, managing the immune system, vision, anti-aging, cancer, macular degeneration, heart health, iron deficiency, inflammation of the joints, diabetes, reducing nausea, and reducing pain for mothers during childbirth, because raspberries prevent hemorrhaging.

Oranges provide nutrients like Vitamin C, A, and B1, beta carotene, pectin, folic acid, calcium, iron, manganese, chlorine and zinc. The antioxidant qualities of this citrus fruit are instrumental in preventing some types of cancer, lowering cholesterol and high blood pressure, strengthening your immune system, easing arthritis, helping regulate the heart, and keeps sperm healthy so it is less likely to cause birth defects in the unborn child. Oranges help to prevent kidney stones, helps with weight loss, prevents ulcers, keeps your teeth and bones strong, and helps to relieve infections and constipation.

Red Grapes, Apple, Cucumber and Mint Vitamin Water

This recipe can be added to your daily vitamin water intake with or without the mint leaves. Throughout the year, I've discovered that red grapes, apples, cucumbers, limes, and certainly mint, are readily available at most local grocery stores. Organic apples are best, but if you can't find them, or if the price isn't within your budget, you can buy any type of red apples and just remove the peel before adding them to your glass jar.

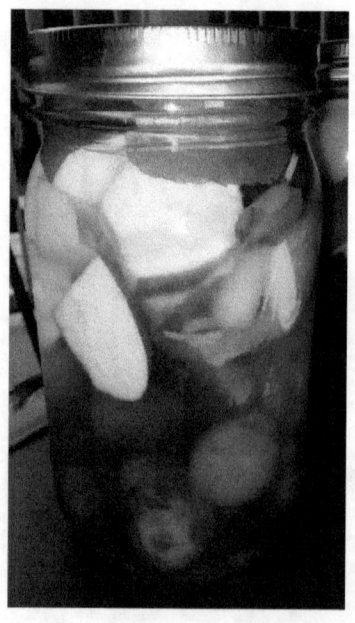

Red grapes, Apple, Mint, and Cucumber Vitamin Water

Ingredients

8-10 red grapes

1 small to medium red apple, peel removed, and chopped into chunks

4-6 inches of cucumber (peeled and sliced)

1/2 fresh lime

4-6 fresh mint leaves, (adjust quantity based on your preference for mint flavor)

Directions

Add the mint leaves to a 1-quart glass jar, and muddle the leaves into the bottom of the jar to extract the mint oil. Add grapes, apple slices, cucumber slices and half of a gently squeezed lime.

Add a handful of ice cubes, fill the jar with water, and seal the jar with a lid. Place in the refrigerator for a minimum of three hours or overnight to allow the water to become infused with the ingredients.

To drink, shake the glass jar to mix up the ingredients with the vitamin water. Then place a small strainer over a drinking glass and pour in your fresh vitamin water mixture.

TIP: If you own a high-speed blender, you can pour the fruits, vegetables, and herbs from the infused water into your blender to make another tasty beverage for later in the day. I don't like to waste food, so by blending the leftover ingredients, I'm getting more vitamins into my body, and I don't have to toss anything into the trash or disposal.

Health Benefits

Mint leaves are known to reduce pain, to help with digestion of fats, and to soothe and calm the stomach.

Apples have so many claims to health fame that people seeking good health probably ignore what they were told growing up. I know that the health and nutrition properties in apples are a *vital* part of my daily diet, and here's why. Apples help you avoid getting Alzheimer's disease, and they protect you from Parkinson's disease. They reduce tooth decay and bacteria in your mouth. They reduce the risk of getting pancreatic cancer by up to 23%. They reduce your chances of getting diabetes, they reduce your bad cholesterol levels, and they make you have a healthier heart. They prevent the formation of gallstones. They help you not get constipated, but they also help if you get diarrhea.

Apples neutralize your system if you have irritable bowel syndrome, and they ward off hemorrhoids. Apples help to control your weight, they boost your immune system, help prevent cataracts, and they detoxify your liver.

Cucumbers are excellent for assisting with hydration, fighting cancer, skin care, blood pressure, teeth and gums, strong nails and hair, relieves arthritis pain, known to cure bad breath, good for those with diabetes, acts as a diuretic, helpful for weight loss, and for promoting hair growth.

Red grapes contain a high water content, which means when ingested, they help to keep your body hydrated. Grapes are a nutrient dense berry with very few calories, and they're ranked high on the antioxidant scale for protecting your body from several types of chronic disease and harmful medical conditions. Grapes can help protect your body from cancer, heart disease, high blood pressure, allergies and constipation.

Limes are great as a thirst-quencher and they contain more vitamin C than a lemon. When you're starting to fall asleep during the day, lime juice helps to keep you awake. It gets rid of those tired and can't-do-anything-today feelings from exhaustion and burnout. Doctors often prescribe that patients consume lime juice to help them lower blood cholesterol, to maintain healthy teeth, gums, and bones, and the vitamin C is known to help resist disease. The rind contains an oil that improves digestion. The juice of a lime helps with constipation, cataracts, and relieves peptic ulcers. Finally, lime juice is known to protect people from bacterial poisoning. For one small, green fruit, this one sure delivers a multitude of health benefits.

Strawberry and Blackberry Vitamin Water

Sometimes, you might have only two fruits available in your kitchen, such as blackberries and strawberries. That's when this two-ingredient recipe comes in handy and is quick to assemble.

Ingredients

6 fresh strawberries, cut in half

1/2 cup blackberries (rinsed), fresh or thawed from frozen

Filtered water

Ice cubes

Directions

Place blackberries into a one-quart glass jar and muddle the berries to extract their juices. Now place the strawberry slices into the jar.

Pour the filtered water over the fruit, add a handful of ice cubes, and seal the glass jar with a lid. Make sure to

allow about one-half inch of space between the
ingredients and the lid.

Health Benefits

Blackberries are such a delicious fruit. In the Pacific
Northwest where I live, they grow wild, and on my daily
walk in spring and summer, I love to stop and pick a few
berries off the branches. Yum! As far as health benefits,
blackberries are at the top of the list of fruits that contain
antioxidants. They help to prevent heart disease as well
as cancer.

If you're having memory problems, blackberries come
to the rescue! They help with memory retention and
hypertension. They improve eyesight, make your blood
vessels stronger, reduce inflammation of intestines, and
they are known to reduce hemorrhoids and upset
stomachs. Plus, blackberries are high in Vitamin C,
Vitamin E, Vitamin A, Vitamin K, fiber, and
Manganese. If you're on the verge of becoming a
diabetic, blackberries lower the risk of you getting
diabetes. They fight obesity, they taste good, they're
available all year long, and when infused in a jar of
vitamin water, they're a definite boost to your health.

Strawberries, regardless if they are fresh or frozen,
contain iodine and antioxidants, such as Vitamin C, that
prevents wrinkles, helps people with thyroid problems,

and regulates your digestive system. Strawberries are an anti-inflammatory, known to prevent cancer and restore eyes to a healthy state, boosts your immune system, assists with the prevention of cardiovascular conditions and improves the health of your bones.

Strawberries, Oranges, and Kiwi Vitamin Water

Sometimes, you might have only three fruits available in your kitchen, such as strawberries, oranges, and kiwi. That's when this three-ingredient recipe comes in handy and is quick to assemble.

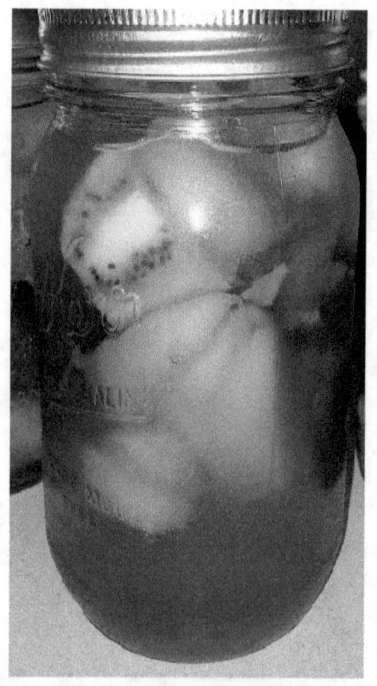

Strawberry, Orange, and Kiwi Vitamin Water

Ingredients

6 fresh strawberries, cut in half

1 Kiwi fruit, peeled and cut in slices

1/4 small orange, cut into slices

Filtered water

Ice cubes

Directions

Place the strawberries into a one-quart glass jar and muddle the berries to extract their juices. Now place the kiwi slices and orange slices into the jar.

Pour the filtered water over the fruit, add a handful of ice cubes, and seal the glass jar with a lid. Make sure to allow about one-half inch of space between the ingredients and the lid.

Health Benefits

Kiwi or Kiwifruit is considered to be a nutrient dense food because its nutrient levels are high, but the fruit contains very few calories. When you add Kiwi to your vitamin water, over time, you will notice that your skin takes on a healthier glow and texture.

Besides making you look good from the inside out, this fruit will help to reduce your blood pressure, and it's been known to lower your chances of suffering from a heart attack and stroke. In addition, the Kiwi has one of the highest levels of vitamin C as compared to other

fruits, and it contains fiber, iron, vitamin A, and potassium; this is quite a powerful vitamin-packed fruit, given its small size. And finally, if you're having trouble getting to sleep or staying asleep at night, the Kiwifruit is said to provide better and improved sleep quality in most adults.

Strawberries, regardless if they are fresh or frozen, contain iodine and antioxidants, such as Vitamin C, that prevents wrinkles, helps people with thyroid problems, regulates your digestive system, is an anti-inflammatory, known to prevent cancer and restore eyes to a healthy state, boosts your immune system, assists with the prevention of cardiovascular conditions and improves the health of your bones.

Oranges provide nutrients like Vitamin C, A, and B1, beta carotene, pectin, folic acid, calcium, iron, manganese, chlorine and zinc. The antioxidant qualities of this citrus fruit are instrumental in preventing some types of cancer, lowering cholesterol and high blood pressure, strengthening your immune system, easing arthritis, helping regulate the heart, and keeps sperm healthy so it is less likely to cause birth defects in the unborn child. Oranges help to prevent kidney stones, helps with weight loss, prevents ulcers, keeps your teeth and bones strong, and helps to relieve infections and constipation.

Strawberry, Lime, and Mint Vitamin Water

Are you suffering from a vitamin deficiency? Instead of taking vitamin supplements, why not prepare your own vitamin water at home? It's simple. It takes only a few minutes. It saves you money!

Ingredients

6 fresh strawberries, cut in half

1 lime, thinly sliced; do not remove the peel

12 fresh mint leaves, chopped fine

Filtered water

Ice cubes

Directions

Start by filling a 1-quart glass jar half full with filtered water, mineral water, or tap water.

Add the six strawberries to the water. With a muddler or wooden spoon, crush the berries. Cut the lime into thin slices and add them to the jar. You can then chop the mint leaves as finely as possible and add them. The mint leaves will make the vitamin water taste even better so you can add as many as you want. Add a handful of ice cubes, fill the jar with water to bring it to within one-half inch of the lid and then seal the jar.

Put the glass jar in the refrigerator overnight. This will give the ingredients plenty of time to release their nutrients and vitamins. You can drink the vitamin water the very next day. It should stay fresh for two to three days as long as you keep the jar refrigerated.

Health Benefits

Mint leaves are known to reduce pain, to help with digestion of fats, and to soothe and calm the stomach.

Limes are great as a thirst-quencher and they contain more vitamin C than a lemon. When you're starting to fall asleep during the day, lime juice helps to keep you awake. It gets rid of those tired and can't-do-anything-today feelings from exhaustion and burnout. Doctors often prescribe that patients consume lime juice to help them lower blood cholesterol, to maintain healthy teeth, gums, and bones, and the vitamin C is known to help resist disease. The rind contains an oil that improves digestion. The juice of a lime helps with constipation, cataracts, and relieves peptic ulcers. Finally, lime juice is known to protect people from bacterial poisoning. For one small, green fruit, this one sure delivers a multitude of health benefits.

Strawberries, regardless if they are fresh or frozen, contain iodine and antioxidants, such as Vitamin C, that prevents wrinkles, helps people with thyroid problems, regulates your digestive system, is an anti-inflammatory, known to prevent cancer and restore eyes to a healthy state, boosts your immune system, assists with the prevention of cardiovascular conditions and improves the health of your bones.

Organic Super Fruit Blend-Veggie Vitamin Water

While I fully endorse buying and using organic fruits, vegetables, and herbs when making vitamin water, today, I discovered a real treat at my local Costco store: Organic Super Fruit Blend. When I saw the packaging and read the ingredient list, I knew that I wanted to turn this bag of organic yumminess into a vitamin water recipe. The organic super fruit blend contains strawberries, cherries, blackberries, blueberries, and pomegranate seeds. You can also buy these fresh super fruits at your local market, and you can find individual bags in the frozen fruit section of your grocery retailer.

Before introducing you to the recipe and prep instructions for creating the vitamin water, I just want to mention that whenever you see assorted varieties of fruits that are packaged together, you can create delicious and healthy vitamin water without having to peel, slice, or clean the fruit. Frozen fruits, when used in fruit-infused vitamin water recipes are just as nutritious as buying fresh fruits.

TIP: These fruits are called super fruits due to their high nutritional value and health benefits. When these fresh fruits are not in season, you can still benefit from buying the frozen variety.

Ingredients

1 cup organic super fruits (thawed from frozen or fresh)

4 - six-inch slices of cucumber (peel removed)

Filtered water

Ice cubes

Directions

Add one cup total of sliced organic super fruits (strawberries, cherries, blackberries, blueberries, and pomegranate seeds), muddled in the bottom of a 1-quart glass jar. To this mixture, add the cucumber slices.

Add a handful of ice cubes to the jar, and fill with water to approximately one-half inch below the rim of the jar. Seal jar, and place in the refrigerator overnight.

To drink the next day, strain the super fruits and cucumber and add the infused vitamin water to a drinking glass or mug. Enjoy!

Health Benefits

Strawberries, regardless if they are fresh or frozen, contain iodine and antioxidants, such as Vitamin C, that prevents wrinkles, helps people with thyroid problems, regulates your digestive system, is an anti-inflammatory, known to prevent cancer and restore eyes to a healthy state, boosts your immune system, assists with the prevention of cardiovascular conditions and improves the health of your bones.

Cherries are a powerful super fruit that provide antioxidant protection, cancer prevention properties, such as fiber, vitamin C, carotenoids and anthocyanins, and cherries are known to reduce effects from gout and inflammation. When the body's uric acid (in your blood) doesn't do its job, you might feel stiffness in your joints or pain from the swelling. Cherries help to relieve all these symptoms and can provide much-needed relief for arthritis and osteoarthritis, too. And what you might not know is that cherries help to reduce belly fat, muscle pain, and they can even lower your risk of a stroke.

Blackberries are such a delicious fruit. In the Pacific Northwest where I live, they grow wild and on my daily walk, I love to stop and pick a few off the braches. Yum! As far as health benefits, blackberries are at the top of the list of fruits that contain antioxidants. They help to prevent heart disease as well as cancer.

If you're having memory problems, blackberries come to the rescue! They help with memory retention and hypertension. They improve eyesight, make your blood vessels stronger, reduce inflammation of intestines, and they are known to reduce hemorrhoids and upset stomachs. Plus, blackberries are high in Vitamin C, Vitamin E, Vitamin A, Vitamin K, fiber, and Manganese. If you're on the verge of becoming a diabetic, blackberries lower the risk of you getting diabetes. They fight obesity, they taste good, they're available all year long, and when infused in a jar of vitamin water, they're a definite boost to your health.

Blueberries provide vitamin C and antioxidants. Also known to improve memory, and they have a favorable impact on blood sugar regulation in persons already diagnosed with type 2 diabetes. In addition, blueberries contain vitamin K, manganese, fiber, and copper.

Pomegranates are high in fiber, low in calories, high in vitamins and phytochemicals, and all this keeps your heart healthy. Plus, this fruit is known to prevent cancer. If you want to lose weight, pomegranate seeds have only 83 calories in about three-quarters of a cup.

Cucumbers are excellent for assisting with hydration, fighting cancer, skin care, blood pressure, teeth and gums, strong nails and hair, relieves arthritis pain, known to cure bad breath, good for those with diabetes, acts as a diuretic, helpful for weight loss, and for promoting hair growth.

Watermelon, Berries, and Lime Vitamin Water

Drinking homemade vitamin water is an excellent way to add more vitamins to your diet. Besides that fact, homemade vitamin water does not contain any preservatives, calories, or added sugar.

You can mix your vitamin water in a 1-quart glass jar and store it in your refrigerator for whenever you need to hydrate your body with water within two to three days. Since you will not be ingesting preservatives into your body, the vitamin water will stay fresh for a couple of days in your refrigerator.

CAUTION: Do not prepare more than four quarts for consumption the next day unless you want to make enough vitamin water for the entire family. For optimum freshness, only store refrigerated quarts of homemade vitamin water for two days.

Ingredients

1 cup watermelon, cubed

1 cup blackberries, crushed or muddled

1 cup strawberries or raspberries, crushed or muddled

1 small lemon or lime, sliced (do not peel)

4 mint leaves, chopped

Filtered water

Ice cubes

Directions

Cut a slice of watermelon and dice it. Add a cup of watermelon cubes into a 1-quart glass jar. Slightly crush a cup of blackberries and strawberries or raspberries depending on what you like best and add it to the glass jar.

Cut a lemon or a lime into thin slices and add it to the glass jar. If you enjoy mint, add three or four chopped mint leaves, add a handful of ice cubes, and fill the jar with water.

Refrigerate the glass jar overnight, remembering that fruits, veggies, and herbs need time to release their vitamins and minerals into the water.

Health Benefits

Watermelons are classified in the same family as cantaloupe, pumpkin, cucumber, and squash. A watermelon contains about 91 percent water by its weight, and it's definitely a thirst quencher. Here are some of the health benefits: improves potency in men, helps prevent heart disease, takes pain away from sore muscles, contains vitamin C, which is an antioxidant, improves your eyesight, helps with immune system deficiencies, and protects against cancer.

And here we just thought it was a fun fruit to bring along on a picnic! You might look at watermelons differently knowing how nutritious they are for your health.

NOTE: It's best to store your uncut watermelon at room temperature rather than putting it in the refrigerator. A room-temperature watermelon contains double the levels of beta carotene, which is a source of vitamin A, and it also contains more lycopene.

Blackberries are such a delicious fruit. In the Pacific Northwest where I live, they grow wild and on my daily walk, I love to stop and pick a few off the braches. Yum! As far as health benefits, blackberries are at the top of the list of fruits that contain antioxidants. They help to prevent heart disease as well as cancer.

If you're having memory problems, blackberries come to the rescue! They help with memory retention and hypertension. They improve eyesight, make your blood vessels stronger, reduce inflammation of intestines, and they are known to reduce hemorrhoids and upset stomachs. Plus, blackberries are high in Vitamin C, Vitamin E, Vitamin A, Vitamin K, fiber, and Manganese.

If you're on the verge of becoming a diabetic, blackberries lower the risk of you getting diabetes. They fight obesity, they taste good, they're available all year long, and when infused in a jar of vitamin water, they're a definite boost to your health.

Mint leaves are known to reduce pain, to help with digestion of fats, and to soothe and calm the stomach.

Limes are great as a thirst-quencher and they contain more vitamin C than a lemon. When you're starting to fall asleep during the day, lime juice helps to keep you awake. It gets rid of those tired and can't-do-anything-today feelings from exhaustion and burnout. Doctors often prescribe that patients consume lime juice to help them lower blood cholesterol, to maintain healthy teeth, gums, and bones, and the vitamin C is known to help resist disease. The rind contains an oil that improves digestion. The juice of a lime helps with constipation, cataracts, and relieves peptic ulcers. Finally, lime juice is known to protect people from bacterial poisoning. For one small, green fruit, this one sure delivers a multitude of health benefits.

Strawberries, regardless if they are fresh or frozen, contain iodine and antioxidants, such as Vitamin C, that prevents wrinkles, helps people with thyroid problems, regulates your digestive system, is an anti-inflammatory, known to prevent cancer and restore eyes to a healthy state, boosts your immune system, assists with the prevention of cardiovascular conditions and improves the health of your bones.

Add Your Notes Here

For quick reference, you might want to list those vitamin water recipes that are known to provide healing remedies for any symptoms or ailments you want to treat.

Conclusion

Thank you again for downloading my book!

I hope you've enjoyed learning about all these great herbs, fruits, and vegetables and how they can restore and protect your health just by adding them to your next glass of water.

Once you begin making your own vitamin water, don't hesitate to experiment. You will quickly discover so many different combinations of fruits, vegetables, and herbs that will be pleasing to the taste, and beneficial for improving your health.

Remember: Natural homemade vitamin water has NO CALORIES and no harsh chemicals or sugars!

Here's to your good health!

Finally, if you liked the recipes and information in this book, take the time to share your thoughts and post a review on the **Amazon website**.

Thank you and good luck!

Ginger Langley

Review this book!

Please leave a review and let me know what you liked about this book by typing the web link below into your favorite browser.

http://www.amazon.com/Vitamin-Water-Recipes-Homemade-Vegetables-ebook/dp/B00J2F8DU8

About the Author

Ginger Langley lives in the Seattle, Washington area, and she loves to cook and experiment with new healthy recipes.

Don't forget to check out her other bestselling books on Amazon:

Coconut Oil Cookbook: Quick and Easy Recipes for Busy Women Who Want to Eat Healthy

Juicing Recipes for Weight Loss, Vitality and Health

Organic Skin Care Recipes for Beginners: Easy and Simple Instructions for Natural Remedies

Coconut Milk Recipes: 21 Quick & Easy Meals for the Busy Professional

Contact Ginger

If you have any questions, or if you have a story you'd like to share about how vitamin water improved your well-being, you can contact me at gingerlangley1@gmail.com.